The 5-Minutes DIY Homemade Hand Sanitizer

A Step by Step Guide on How to Use Natural Essential Oils to Make Your Own Hand Sanitizer Gel and Spray Recipes to Protect Yourself From Bacteria and Viruses

By

Dr. Lee Henton

Copyright © 2020 – Dr. Lee Henton

All rights reserved

No part of this publication may be reproduced, distributed, or transmitted in any form or by any means, including photocopying, recording, or other electronic or mechanical methods, without the prior written permission of the publisher, except in the case of brief quotations embodied in reviews and certain other non-commercial uses permitted by copyright law.

Disclaimer

This publication is designed to provide reliable information on the subject matter only for educational purposes, and it is not intended to provide medical advice for any medical treatment. You should always consult your doctor or physician for guidance before you stop, start, or alter any prescription medications or attempt to implement the methods discussed. This book is published independently by the author and has no affiliation with any brands or products mentioned within it. The author hereby disclaims any responsibility or liability whatsoever that is incurred from the use or application of the contents of this publication by the purchaser or reader. The purchaser or reader is hereby responsible for his or her own actions.

Table of Contents

About The Author..5

Introduction..6

Chapter 1..10

The ABC of Hand Sanitizers...10

    Hand Sanitizer and Its Importance.................................11

    Hand Sanitizers Vs. Hand Washing................................12

    Alcohol-Based Sanitizers Vs. Alcohol-Free Sanitizers........14

    Effectiveness of Hand Sanitizers Against Germs..............15

        What Germs Can Alcohol-Based Hand Sanitizer Kill? . 16

    DIY Hand Sanitizer Benefits..19

    Are DIY Hand Sanitizers Safe?......................................22

Chapter 2..25

Making Homemade Sanitizers...25

    Hand Sanitizer Tools You Need to Have.........................25

    Hand Sanitizer Ingredients You Need to Get...................28

        Isopropyl (Rubbing Alcohol) or Ethanol........................29

        Aloe Vera Gel 29

Essential Oils..30

Hand Sanitizer Ingredient You Must Not Use................32

Vodka..32

Witch Hazel 33

Safety Precautions for Making Your Hand Sanitizers.......35

Recipes For Homemade Hand Sanitizers......................37

The WHO Hand Sanitizer Formula 38

Simple Standard Hand Sanitizer 40

Vitamin E Oil Hand Sanitizer 41

Kid-Friendly Hand Sanitizers By Age Group 42

Citrus Mint Hand Sanitizer 43

Lavender-Tea Tree "Little Tykes" Hand Sanitizer 44

Thieves Hand Sanitizer 45

Glycerin-Based Hand Sanitizer... 46

Chapter 3..50

Hand Hygiene Practice...50

Why Is It important?...50

Handwashing the Right Way....................................51

Using Hand Sanitizers Effectively............................53

Conclusion..55

References..58

About The Author

Dr. Lee Henton is a US-trained General Practice Doctor from the Johns Hopkins University School of Medicine with additional qualification in nutritional medicine from Iowa State University. He is a certified specialist in dietology and nutrition.

He has extensive years of medical and nutritional experience across general medicine, pediatrics, traumatology, addictions, food nutrition, and diet therapy.

He currently runs a co-established private medical and wellness practice where he operates from. His approach is personalized with each client by combining medical and food nutrition counseling. All advice he provides is at par with his experience, as well as with medical and nutritional concepts. He specializes primarily in men and women's health.

He lives in Minnesota with his wife and two daughters.

Introduction

Since the outbreak of COVID-19, sales of hand sanitizers have soared tremendously, resulting in not only its scarcity but also the unnecessary increase in its cost of purchase virtually in most online stores, pharmacies, and supermarkets. This is exactly what happens when the demand exceeds the supply.

According to the World Health Organization (WHO) and U.S. Centers for Disease Control and Prevention (CDC), hand washing is by far the most effective way to not only destroy the coronavirus but also protect yourself from most bacteria and viruses, while recommending that hand sanitizers be used only when hand washing is practically unforeseeable. Hand sanitizers with an alcohol concentration of 60% and above are recognized by WHO and CDC as very effective in destroying most germs, which includes the coronavirus; however, not all commercially sold hand sanitizers are made effective against this virus, and most likely, against other bacteria and viruses because of the lower concentration of alcohol it contains. This has made homemade hand sanitizers much more appealing, where buying at an overpriced amount can finally be averted, but most importantly, where greater control over the ingredients and the quality of the hand sanitizer can be exercised. With that being said, making your own hand sanitizer is not a walk in the park, especially for an average consumer who knows nothing about the right ingredients to use, the safety precautions that must be adhered to, and the ratio of alcohol to ingredients that must be followed to produce the final 60% and above concentration. It could be a mess if you don't get this right. Not to worry, this book is designed to take you through each step of the process on the dos and don'ts of making your own hand sanitizer at home. And not just that, this book uses an easy to understand language with little to no scientific jargon, even if you don't have a background in science.

At the end of this book, you will:

- Gain a deeper understanding of how hand sanitizers work against bacteria and viruses such

as coronavirus, its importance, and its dos and don'ts.
- Be enlightened on why alcohol-based hand sanitizers should be used over alcohol-free hand sanitizers.
- Know the type of germs alcohol-based hand sanitizers can destroy and what type it cannot destroy.
- Understand the real benefits of making your own hand sanitizer.
- Know why you must not use certain ingredients recommended over the internet to make your own hand sanitizer.
- Uncover all you need to get started in making your own hand sanitizer, thereby subtracting the noise and inconsistencies all over the internet.
- Be well educated on the important safety precautions you must adhere to when making your own hand sanitizer.
- Be familiar with the necessary tools, ingredients, and steps you need to follow to make your own WHO and CDC recommended hand sanitizer.

- Know how to prepare several homemade hand sanitizer recipes in 5 minutes, using the right alcohol proportion and different essential oil ingredients that are both safe for your kids, families, and friends and effective against most bacteria and viruses, e.g., coronavirus.
- Be better informed on when to wash your hands over when to use hand sanitizers against germs.
- Understand what hand hygiene entails, its importance and how to apply it correctly during hand washing and usage of hand sanitizers against germs

…And much more.

So, without further ado, let's begin proper.

Chapter 1

The ABC of Hand Sanitizers

Hand sanitizers were developed for use after handwashing or for times when there is no availability of soap and water.

If you have been in a child's play area, then you must have witnessed how mothers reach for their purse to grab their hand sanitizers as their children come off the play equipment, where each child is given a dab of sanitizer to rub against their hands to disinfect the germs transferred to their skin – in the hope that this practice keeps the children, and their families healthier. Or is it one of those days in late fall when you are stuck at home and covered in each blanket you own, downing bowl after bowl of soup, then having to regret every handshake you gave over the past week, wishing you took necessary steps to put an effective hand sanitizing procedure in place. Well, with the current global pandemic, that time has come for you to put a touchpoint cleaning procedure in place such as handwashing and sanitizing procedures.

Hand Sanitizer and Its Importance

Hand sanitizers, also referred to as hand rub is a liquid or gel that is applied to the hands to destroy common pathogens or infectious agents or simply, germs, i.e., disease-causing micro-organisms such as virus and bacteria.

In general,

- Hand sanitizers are not only convenient and portable especially when we are unable to wash our hands with soap and water whenever we need to disinfect our hands, but they are also easy to use
- Several studies show that there is a reduced risk of spreading gastrointestinal (stomach) and respiratory infection (e.g., influenza) among families who use hand sanitizers
- Most commercially made hand sanitizers (alcohol and alcohol-free) are made up of compounds

such as glycerol that help prevent skin dryness and irritation.

Hand Sanitizers Vs. Hand Washing

Hand sanitizers provide an effective and convenient way through which your hands can be cleaned if soap and water are not available, and your hands are not covered with visible dirt, grease, or chemicals such as pesticides and heavy metals. A 2019 ruling by the Food and Drug Administration (FDA) states that a product can be referred to as a hand sanitizer if it is made up of ethyl alcohol (alternatively called ethanol), Isopropyl alcohol (isopropanol) or benzalkonium chloride as the active ingredient. Any other ingredients that do not comprise these three have shown little to no evidence of being effective at killing germs and have not won the approval of the FDA.

Nonetheless, when it comes to preventing the spread of infectious diseases such as the infamous COVID-19, really and truly, nothing beats the good old-fashioned method of handwashing. Knowing when best to wash your hands, and when to turn to hand sanitizers is vital to protecting yourself not only from the novel coronavirus but other illnesses such as the common cold and seasonal flu (e.g., influenza A virus). The US Centers for Disease Control and Prevention (CDC) and the WHO recommends that whenever possible, handwashing with soap and water should be adopted as the first line of defense against germs because it helps destroy the amount of all types of germs found on the hands. However, if soap and water are not readily available or accessible, and your hands are not covered with visible dirt, grease, or chemicals, the next best option, according to CDC and WHO is using a hand sanitizer with an alcohol concentration of at least 60 percent – this not only kills the germs (including the coronaviruses) but also helps prevent its spread to others. However, not all types of germs are destroyed even with a hand sanitizer of 60 percent alcohol or above. For certain types of germs such as norovirus (not to be confused with coronavirus), Cryptosporidium (a parasite that can cause diarrhea), and Clostridium difficile (a bacteria that causes bowel and diarrhea problems), studies show that handwashing is much effective in removing such germs than using hand sanitizers.

Alcohol-Based Sanitizers Vs. Alcohol-Free Sanitizers

Depending on the active ingredient used, hand sanitizers are classified as either alcohol-based or alcohol-free sanitizers.

- Alcohol-based sanitizers are unarguably known to kill most micro-organisms or germs. Alcohol-based sanitizers are primarily made up of about 60% to 95% alcohol, usually in the form of ethanol, isopropanol, or n-propanol. At these concentrations of alcohol, the protein (which is vital for the survival and multiplication of micro-organisms) composition in certain micro-organisms is immediately destroyed, thus effectively neutralizing the micro-organisms.

  Hand sanitizers below 60 percent of alcohol are found only to reduce the growth of germs and are less effective at destroying it.

- Alcohol-free sanitizers are primarily disinfectants-based, which contains the quaternary ammonium compounds (usually the benzalkonium chloride) or anti-microbial agents, such as triclosan instead of alcohol. Although this can reduce the amount of micro-organisms on the hands, it is, however, less effective than the alcohol-based sanitizers when it comes to destroying micro-organisms.

Effectiveness of Hand Sanitizers Against Germs

Although variability in the efficacy of hand sanitizers are prevalent given that not all hand sanitizers are made equally, hand sanitizers nonetheless can help control how infectious diseases are transmitted, especially in situations where there is poor compliance with handwashing. Agencies such as the WHO and CDC promotes the use of alcohol-based hand sanitizers over alcohol-free hand sanitizers due to the safety concerns about the chemicals used in the production of alcohol-free products. Study shows that certain anti-microbial compounds, for example, triclosan which is used in the production of alcohol-free hand sanitizers may interfere with the functioning of the endocrine system. Based on the mounting concerns over triclosan in 2014, authorities in the European Union (E.U.) thus had to limit its usage in several consumer products across the E.U. member countries. Not only that, alcohol-free disinfectants and antimicrobials can also potentially result in the development of anti-microbial resistance, thus making alcohol-free sanitizers less effective in destroying germs.

In subsequent sections of this book, I would focus only on alcohol-based hand sanitizers and how it can be prepared to satisfy the required alcohol volume or concentration.

What Germs Can Alcohol-Based Hand Sanitizer Kill?

According to the CDC, an alcohol-based hand sanitizer that satisfies the alcohol volume or concentration requirement can not only reduce the amount of microbes (same as micro-organisms or germs) on your hands but also help destroy a variety of disease-causing agents or pathogens on your hands, such as the SARS-CoV-2 (severe acute respiratory coronavirus 2), colloquially known as coronavirus or COVID-19. Alcohol-based hand sanitizers are also effective at killing many types of bacteria, which include but are not limited to:

- Methicillin-Resistant Staphylococcus Aureus (MRSA), an infection caused by the Staphylococcus bacteria and resistant to many antibiotics, and;
- Escherichia coli (a bacterium that can produce bloody diarrhea).

Also, alcohol-based hand sanitizers are effective in destroying many viruses, including the hepatitis A virus, Middle East respiratory syndrome coronavirus (MERS-CoV), rhinovirus, HIV, and the influenza A virus.

However, certain types of germs cannot be destroyed by even the best alcohol-based hand sanitizers, most notably:

- Norovirus
- Cryptosporidium and;
- Clostridium difficile (also known as C. diff)

Nonetheless, the effectiveness of alcohol-based hand sanitizers in destroying germs relies on many factors, vis-à-vis how it is applied (e.g., the quantity used, the length of exposure, the frequency of use), and whether the particular infectious agents found on the hands are susceptible to the active ingredient of the hand sanitizer. The general rule of thumb of alcohol-based hand sanitizers requires that it is rubbed thoroughly over the surfaces of the finger and hand for at least 30 seconds, followed by total air-drying. In addition, hand sanitizers may not work properly if your hands are visibly dirty or greasy. In such a case, you should opt for handwashing instead of hand sanitizer.

Also, bear in mind that hand sanitizers do expire, which by industry-standard is about two to three years from the date of production if kept in proper condition; this is because when the alcohol in the mixture evaporates over a while, and if it goes below 60 percent, the solution becomes ineffective against germs.

DIY Hand Sanitizer Benefits

There is no doubt that some commercial hand sanitizers do their job in destroying germs such as bacteria and viruses; however, not all commercial hand sanitizers are effective enough in destroying germs. As a matter of fact, some commercial hand sanitizers are made up of as little as 57% alcohol, thus making homemade products more suitable to opt for, especially if done right. Also, a good hand sanitizer should contain other ingredients that can hydrate your skin, but in all honesty, do we really take note of each word written on commercial product labels? And to be frank, when armed with the right knowledge in making homemade sanitizers especially in times of scarcity of commercial hand sanitizers, you become more cautious and aware of what to do and not do when making your own hand sanitizers; giving you more independent control in making hand sanitizers that can not only match that obtained in some commercial products but also exceed their effectiveness. That being said, let's briefly have a look at some of the common benefits of homemade sanitizers.

More quantity

Conventionally, most commercial hand sanitizers are sold in small bottles. If used frequently, it may run out before you know it, thus making homemade sanitizers more preferable since it affords you the ability to produce how much quantity you deem desirable to meet your needs and those of your families.

Saves money

Being able to make your own hand sanitizer and reuse the bottle allows you to minimize unnecessary expenditures when making a new one.

Ingredient management

As earlier mentioned, we can't be all too sure or trusting of the quality of ingredients that are used in most commercial hand sanitizing products, making homemade products more desirable to opt for since it allows us to control what compound goes into it.

Scent option

One of the benefits of homemade hand sanitizers is that it allows you to customize the scent of the essential oils to your desired flavor, especially if you are allergic or sensitive to certain scents, or you can leave them out completely.

Chemical-free

Most commercial based hand sanitizers are produced using chemical compounds that have been found to either be ineffective against the coronavirus or harmful to the body. One of such compound is the triclosan chemical compound which has been flagged by the FDA as a compound not to be used for over the counter consumer products given its potential potency to cause abnormal endocrine system issues. Another of such compound is benzalkonium chloride, an alcohol substitute used in the production of popular alcohol-free hand sanitizer products such as Germ-X and Purell.

However, when it comes to combatting the coronavirus, the CDC notes that this ingredient is less reliable than the alcohol-based products. On the other hand, homemade hand sanitizers do not make use of these chemicals because, with the right knowledge, you are more informed not to include these chemicals when making your own hand sanitizer.

Are DIY Hand Sanitizers Safe?

It's no longer news that hand sanitizers were one of the first products of defense against the global pandemic to have flown off the shelves and is still almost impossible to get any online or in stores. This has resulted in many attempting their own DIY versions using recipes available all over the internet, which begs the question, are homemade hand sanitizers really safe?

Going by medical requirements, making your own hand sanitizer is not recommended partly because a proper hand sanitizer recipe is all about the proportions, which understandably is difficult for an average consumer to get right. When the proportions or ingredients become off in your little homemade laboratory;

- It renders the product as ineffective, meaning the sanitizer may not destroy the risk of exposure to germs
- It can lead to skin irritation, injury, or burns, and;
- You can become exposed to hazardous chemicals through inhalation.

Another big red flag is that the tools being used must also be sanitized, which is the whole point of hand sanitizers, and if you do not correctly sanitize the tools, the potency of the final product could be compromised.

In addition to using correctly sanitized tools, the WHO's hand sanitizer recipe (later discussed in subsequent sections) also requires that production facilities be air-conditioned and flame-free (ethanol and Isopropyl alcohol are extremely flammable).

Thus, the recipes described in this book are intended to be used by professionals possessing both the expertise and the resources to make homemade hand sanitizers safely. Homemade hand sanitizer is only recommended in extreme situations when you are not able to wash your hands with soap and water or for the foreseeable future.

Having pointed out all these vital concerns as to why homemade sanitizers might not be entirely safe, especially if you are defaulting in any of the concerns mentioned, proceeding otherwise to making your own hand sanitizers using the recipes discussed in this book must be done with extreme caution and adherence to all safety practices.

Chapter 2

Making Homemade Sanitizers

In all honesty, making your own hand sanitizer is quick and easy, typically about 5 minutes, especially if you have familiarized yourself with the necessary procedures and precautions to be adhered to. Also, much if not all of the ingredients and tools that you require to get started are available in the personal care section of most grocery stores, such as Whole Foods Market, pharmacy stores, as well as several online retailers, such as Amazon.

Hand Sanitizer Tools You Need to Have

Before you get started in making your own hand sanitizer, it is essential to have the basic tools to facilitate this process. The items below are a worthy investment to make if you don't have them at home.

Mixing Bowl: Required for mixing all your ingredients. Ideally, one that can hold up to three to five cups of liquid would suffice.

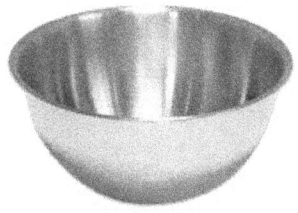

Measuring Spoon: Required when adding a specific or small amount of ingredient to the recipe.

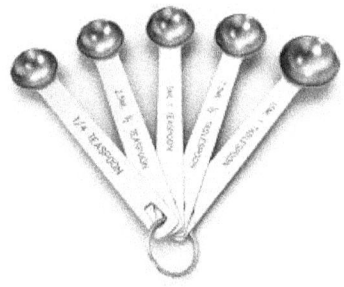

Measuring Cup or Jug: A measuring cup or jug is a container (in glass or plastic) with lines printed on its sides used for measuring liquids, which shows the amount it contains. It is very useful when you need to measure ingredients in cup sizes.

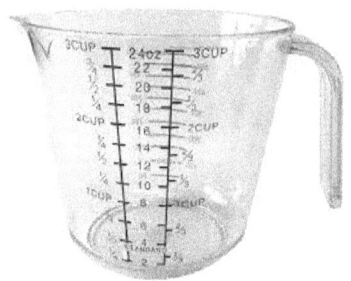

Plastic Funnel: Required to transfer the finished hand-sanitizing product from the bowl into a bottle. Ideally, a small-sized funnel that fits into the bottle would suffice.

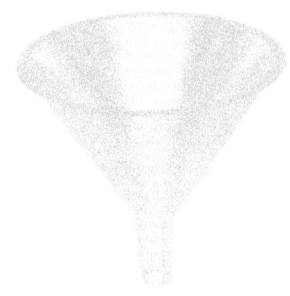

Nitrile Gloves: Required to prevent your hands from being burned when making the hand sanitizer.

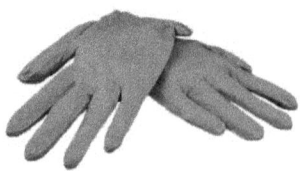

PET Pump or Spray Bottles: Required to store the hand sanitizer once ready. Dark-colored PET pump or spray bottles are most ideal when making your hand sanitizer because when essential oils are added to your hand sanitizer, the dark-colored bottle will prevent degradation of the essential oils from U.V. light.

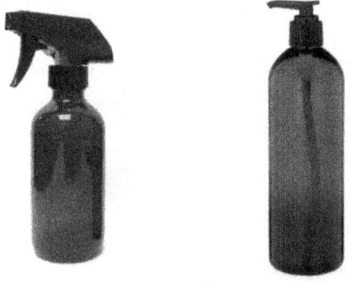

Hand Sanitizer Ingredients You Need to Get

Three main ingredients are typically used when making homemade sanitizer. However, in one or a few recipes I would be discussing shortly, other ingredients may be required either as a substitute to the main ingredient (when the main ingredient is not available) or as an additional ingredient, so be on the lookout for such.

Isopropyl (Rubbing Alcohol) or Ethanol

Isopropyl alcohol or ethanol is the main active ingredient in hand sanitizers, and for your homemade sanitizer to be effective in killing germs, especially the coronaviruses, then you must ensure to use undiluted Isopropyl alcohol that has a concentration of 91% percent or above. Ideally, 99% is a common concentration being used; however, anything above 91% will still be effective in killing germs.

Getting hold of Isopropyl can be difficult to come by; however, in such a case, you can opt for pure ethanol instead. Ethanol is the alcohol found in spirits, and one of such recommended spirits is Everclear (a type of grain alcohol), which should be 190 proof (about 95% alcohol volume) for it to be effective in killing germs.

Aloe Vera Gel

Isopropyl alcohol needs to be mixed with an emollient, such as aloe vera, which is necessary to add moisture to your hands to soften or soothe your skin else, the Isopropyl alcohol will not only dry out your hands but will also get it cracked or burned. The same applies if you don't use enough aloe vera gel; hence, the need to use the right ratio.

Nonetheless, the ratio you need to make an effective germ-busting hand sanitizer relies on the percentage of alcohol used and the most notable ratio is 2:1

For example, if the Isopropyl alcohol you are using has a concentration of 91%, then the ratio of alcohol to aloe vera will be 2:1, e.g., 3 tbsp of alcohol to 1.5 tbsp of aloe vera, or 2 cups of alcohol to 1 cup of aloe vera gel, the same ratio applies when using 99% Isopropyl alcohol.

Vegetable glycerin can also be used in the absence of aloe vera. Both are used as moisturizers for the hands.

Essential Oils

While adding essential oils to your mixture is optional, however, if you detest the smell of alcohol and need to add some fragrance to the mixture that has a germ-busting characteristic, then adding essential oils is your best bet. However, when it comes to hand sanitizers, there a few essential oils amongst the varieties that can be used both as fragrance and germ-busting. One such is the tee tree essential oils, which, by far, is the most recommended essential oil to use for hand sanitizer. According to Medical News Today, the properties of tea tree oil comes with antibacterial features as well as anti-inflammatory, anti-fungal, and antiviral features properties. While there is limited research on the viruses the tea tree essential oil can combat successfully, it is thought to combat the pathogens that are associated with acne, staphylococci, micrococci, Enterococcus faecalis, and Pseudomonas aeruginosa. Lavender, eucalyptus and cinnamon, just like the tee tree, are yet another common essential oil with antiviral, antibacterial, and anti-fungal features. Other popular brands of essential oils are lemon, sweet or wild orange, rosemary, clove, thyme, and peppermint. Whichever type of essential oil you decide to use, caution should be applied because some fragrances could cause an allergic reaction. For example, the lemon essential oil, when used, can cause a phototoxic skin reaction.

Hand Sanitizer Ingredient You Must Not Use

It is a known fact that the internet is awash with several recipes on how to make your own hand sanitizer. However, not all the ingredients being recommended online are ideal for making hand sanitizers, especially if you are out to make a hand sanitizer that can kill the coronaviruses. Two of such commonly recommended ingredients you must not use in making your hand sanitizers are vodka and witch hazel.

Vodka

Vodka is one common ingredient that most recipes for homemade hand sanitizers recommend in the absence of Isopropyl. Most U.S. vodka comes in the standard 80 Proof, which would give about 40% undiluted alcohol concentration. However, some vodka if you can get hold of them also come in 120 proof, about 60% undiluted alcohol concentration, nonetheless, this is still not suitable for use in making your own hand sanitizer especially because you would most likely dilute this concentration with aloe vera, or glycerin which would further reduce the concentration to less than 60% of the

WHO and CDC recommendation. Additionally, the FDA has only approved the use of USP grade ingredients for making hand sanitizers, and vodka is not a USP grade certified alcohol.

Witch Hazel

Witch hazel is a tree-like plant that is indigenous to North America and some parts of Asia. According to the National Institutes of Health (NIH), the extract is gotten from the bark or leaves of the plant and mostly used as an astringent to relieve mild skin irritations such as bites from insect and minor cut or scrapes. This is due to its richness in tannins (compounds found in plants, seeds, bark, and leaves, known to possess some anti-microbial and anti-inflammatory properties), thus its popularity as an ingredient in skincare products.

But does witch hazel actually kill germs?

According to Amesh A. Adalja, a senior scholar of infectious disease at the Johns Hopkins Center for Health Security, "although witch hazel contains chemical compounds that can shrink or constrict body tissues, it is unreliable in killing germs due to the absence of evidence that ascertains its effectiveness as an antiseptic."

This means that witch hazel should not be used as the single germ-bursting ingredient in hand sanitizing solutions, especially those with claims to destroy the coronaviruses, says Rajeev Fernando, M.D., an infectious disease expert in Southampton, New York.

In other words, the many ingredients available on the internet that uses witch hazel in the making of hand sanitizers will not be effective against germs.

Also, the mixing of bleach and ammonia should not be attempted because doing so produces a toxic gas called chloramine, which could lead to chest pain and shortness of breath. Besides, bleach and vinegar should also not be mixed to produce hand sanitizers because it can produce chlorine gas that causes coughing, burning, breathing problems, and watery eyes.

Safety Precautions for Making Your Hand Sanitizers

According to Jagdish Khubchandani, an associate professor of health science at Ball State University, making your hand sanitizer at home requires that you adhere strictly to these tips:

- Hand sanitizers should be made in a clean space, and all countertops should be wiped with a diluted bleach solution prior to the production process.
- Hands must be washed thoroughly before making the hand sanitizer.
- Make use of a clean spoon, mixing bowl, whisk, glass, or spray bottles by washing these items thoroughly before their usage.
- Ensure the alcohol in the final product is not diluted below the recommended 60% concentration
- All ingredients should be thoroughly mixed until they are well blended.
- The mixture should not be touched with your hands until it is ready for use.

- Your homemade production facility or laboratory should be air-conditioned and flame-free (ethanol and Isopropyl alcohol are extremely flammable). Also, if it comes in contact with your hands, it will burn your skin, hence, ensure to wear nitrile gloves.
- All homemade sanitizers should be properly labeled to prevent anyone from mistakenly ingesting it.

A Short message from the Author:

Hey, I hope you are enjoying the book? I would love to hear your thoughts!

Many readers do not know how hard reviews are to come by and how much they help an author.

I would be incredibly grateful if you could take just 60 seconds to write a short review on the product page of this book, even if it is a few sentences!

Thanks for the time taken to share your thoughts!

Your review will genuinely make a difference for me and help gain exposure for my work.

Recipes For Homemade Hand Sanitizers

Besides the alcohol used in each recipe, other ingredients are employed to help moisturize your hands and make it smell nice. Note that the proportion of ingredients used in the recipes below all amounts to a final alcohol content that is around 60% and above, which is the recommendation by the WHO and CDC.

Without further ado, let's proceed.

The WHO Hand Sanitizer Formula

The WHO's recipe for hand sanitizer is primarily used for local production where the production facility is WHO compliant, and not for homemade preparation. However, the recipe below has been scaled down for homemade usage.

To make 1 1/3 cups of hand sanitizer, mix the ingredients below in a mixing bowl that can accommodate three to five cups of liquid

Ingredients:

- 1 cup of 99% Isopropyl alcohol or 1 cup plus 4 teaspoons of 91% Isopropyl alcohol
- 1 tablespoon of 3% hydrogen peroxide (needed to destroy the spores of several bacterias in your ingredients and not on your hands)
- 1 teaspoon of 98% glycerin
- Boiled cold water or sterile distilled water

Directions:

- Pour the alcohol, peroxide, and glycerin into a mixing bowl, then add sufficient water to bring the quantity to a total of 1 1/3 cups. Mix properly.
- Use a funnel to pour the finished sanitizer into a spray bottle and label accordingly.

Note: Because water was used in the preparation, the final product would have less of a gel consistency, hence the need to use a spray bottle.

The final alcohol concentration of this WHO formula is 75%, making it very effective in killing germs such as the novel coronavirus.

Simple Standard Hand Sanitizer

This recipe is one of the most common types of recipes out there, easy to make in no time.

For 91% Isopropyl alcohol:

Ingredients:

- 2/3 cups of 91% Isopropyl alcohol
- 1/3 cup of 100% pure aloe vera gel
- 10 drops of tea tree or lavender essential oil or both

For 99% Isopropyl alcohol:

Ingredients:

- 3/4 cups of 99% Isopropyl alcohol
- 1/4 cup of 100% pure aloe vera gel
- 10 drops of tea tree or lavender essential oil or both

Directions:

Pour the alcohol and the aloe vera gel into a bowl, then add the drops of essential oils. Mix properly using a spoon or spatula.

1. Use a funnel to pour the finished sanitizer into a 2-ounce pump bottle and label accordingly.

Vitamin E Oil Hand Sanitizer

This hand sanitizer recipe is made from ingredients with antibacterial, antiviral, and anti-fungal properties, which are all good for the skin. However, the vitamin E oil used nourishes the skin, keeping it hydrated and clean, and also helps preserve the sanitizer.

Ingredients:

- 12 teaspoons of 190 proof Everclear (95% alcohol) or higher Isopropyl alcohol
- 10 drops of lavender essential oil
- 6 drops of lemongrass essential oil
- 25 drops of tea tree essential oil

- 6 teaspoons of aloe vera gel
- 1 teaspoon of vitamin E oil

Direction:

1. Mix the essential oils and vitamin E oil in a mixing bowl.
2. Pour the alcohol into the mixture and mix, then add the aloe vera gel, mixing properly
3. Transfer the sanitizer to a 2-ounce spray bottle and shake gently before using it. Label accordingly.

Kid-Friendly Hand Sanitizers By Age Group

The essential oils used in this recipe are considered kid-friendly, which is why I am comfortable sharing this recipe with you. If you want a cheap, safe, and effective way of making a homemade essential oil hand sanitizer not only for your children but for yourself, then the recipes shared below is your best bet. Whether it's the season of cold or flu, your kids returning to school, or you simply want to protect yourself and kids from the global coronavirus pandemic, and other germs, the below recipes would serve your kids best.

Citrus Mint Hand Sanitizer

This hand sanitizer recipe uses a mix of antibacterial, antiviral, anti-microbial, and anti-fungal essential oil properties to kill most germs on the hands. This hand sanitizer is appropriate for kids age 10 and up, and should not be used on kids below 10 years old.

Ingredients:

- 4 teaspoon of 190 proof Everclear (95% alcohol)
- 1 tsp of aloe vera gel
- 1 tsp of unscented Castille soap
- 5 drops of rosemary essential oil
- 3 drops of lemon essential oil
- 2 drops of peppermint essential oil

Directions:

1. Fill a 1-ounce spray bottle with the alcohol and essential oils. Shake properly and allow it to sit undisturbed for some hours so that the alcohol can dissolve as many of the essential oils as possible.
2. After a couple of hours, the aloe vera and Castille soap should be added into the spray bottle, cap the bottle, and shake thoroughly. Label accordingly.

Lavender-Tea Tree "Little Tykes" Hand Sanitizer

This hand sanitizer recipe makes use of a mix of two of the most gentle and safest essential oils in a dilution that is appropriate for kids aged 2 – 6 years. This should not be used for kids below 2 years old.

Ingredients:

- 4 teaspoon of 190 proof Everclear (95% alcohol)
- 1 tsp of aloe vera gel
- 1 tsp of unscented Castille soap

- 2 drops of lavender essential oil
- 1 drop of tea tree essential oil

Note: For directions on how to mix, follow the same directions highlighted just above

Thieves Hand Sanitizer

The thieves hand sanitizer below comes in two recipes that are suitable for two categories of age group.

For children 6 months and above:

This hand sanitizer recipe can be used on children aged 6 months and above. It should not be used on children below 6 months.

Ingredients:

- 4 teaspoon of 190 proof Everclear (95% alcohol)
- 1 tsp of aloe vera gel
- 1 tsp of unscented Castille soap
- 5 drops of cinnamon leaf essential oil
- 3 drops of sweet orange essential oil
- 2 drops of pine essential oil

For children 10 years old and above:

This hand sanitizer is for children 10 years old and above. It should not be used on children below 10 years.

Ingredients:

- 4 teaspoons of 190 proof Everclear (95% alcohol)
- 1 tsp of aloe vera gel
- 1 tsp unscented Castille soap
- 6 drops of thieves essential oil blend

Note: For directions on how to mix, follow the same directions highlighted just above.

Glycerin-Based Hand Sanitizer

The essential oils used in this recipe are also considered kid-friendly with glycerin substituting for aloe vera.

Ingredients:

- 3-4 tablespoons of 190 proof Everclear (95% alcohol) or higher Isopropyl alcohol
- 1/2 teaspoon of glycerin

- 20 drops of tea tree essential oil*
- 10 drops of spruce essential oil**
- 6 drops of lemon essential oil***

Direction:

1. Mix the glycerin and the essential oils in a mixing bowl and add it to a 2-ounce spray bottle.
2. Pour in the alcohol to a level where the bottle is almost full, then cover the bottle with its cap and shake properly to combine the ingredients.
3. Gently shake before using it. Label accordingly

Note:

*This is about 2% dilution. A dilution of 5-15% is deemed safe for skincare.

**This is about 1% dilution.

***This is about 0.5% dilution. Dilution below 2% causes no photo-toxicity, with up to 5% dilution considered safe for skincare.

If you don't want to purchase the individual essential oils, you can use a kid-safe essential oil blend, like the Germ Destroyer from Plant Therapy. If you decide to go this route, you would have to follow the dilution direction shared on Plant Therapy's product page at https://www.planttherapy.com/germ-destroyer-kidsafe-essential-oil

The end… almost!

Hey! We've made it to the final chapter of this book, and I hope you've enjoyed it so far.

If you have not done so yet, I would be incredibly thankful if you could take just a minute to leave a quick review on this book's product page.

Reviews are not easy to come by, and as an independent author with a little marketing budget, I rely on you, my readers, to leave a short review on my book.

Even if it is just a sentence or two!

So if you really enjoyed this book, please leave a brief review.

I truly appreciate your effort to leave your review, as it truly makes a huge difference.

Thanks once again from the depth of my heart for purchasing this book and reading it to the end.

Chapter 3

Hand Hygiene Practice

Hand hygiene entails the practice of cleaning your hands with soap and water or with an alcohol-based hand rub, such as hand sanitizer. The purpose of hand hygiene is for the removal of grease, dirt, or other unwanted substances that could result in the spread of many diseases. For example, people can be infected with respiratory diseases such as influenza or the common cold, if for example, they do not wash their hands properly before touching their eyes, nose, or mouth. When performed correctly, hand hygiene results in not only the reduction of micro-organisms or germs on the hands but also destroys many germs that are found on the hands, thus preventing its spread to others.

Why Is It important?

A good hand hygiene practice is one of the most effective ways to prevent the spread of infections such as the coronavirus and other infections earlier discussed in this book. The truth is most infections amongst people are caused by spreading germs from person-to-person. Even though your hands may look clean, they can still be a carrier of germs, and the reason for this is because germs are so small that you won't be able to see them, making it so easy to spread these germs to others without realizing it. That is why washing your hands regularly is highly recommended, not just when it's covered with visible grease or dirt. Using alcohol-based hand sanitizers where water and soap are not immediately accessible is also recommended. However, this should not be used as a substitute for handwashing, which is by far the most effective way to keep your hands free from germs and disease spreading agents.

Handwashing the Right Way

Many of us hardly pay attention to how we wash our hands; still, I get a strong feeling that this narrative is changing maybe as a result of the current global pandemic where proper hand hygiene is being emphasized as very essential to curbing the spread of the virus. It is also noteworthy to mention that your hands should be washed:

- after you cough, sneeze or blow your nose
- before, during and after preparing food
- after going to the toilet or changing a nappy
- when your hands are visibly dirty
- after smoking
- after handling or patting animals
- before and after taking care of someone who is sick
- before eating and;
- after touching surfaces that could be contaminated

This list is not exhaustive; however, depending on your situation, always ensure to wash your hands, make it a ritual.

But most importantly is that the aforementioned be done the right way else it counters the purpose, which is to reduce and destroy the germs on your hands and curtail its spread to others. To this effect, the CDC has released a guideline with specific instructions on the most effective way to wash your hands. This is what they recommend:

1. Always make use of clean, running water
2. Washing your hands with warm water and soap is the gold standard for hand hygiene, as well as preventing the spread of infectious diseases. When the hands are washed with warm water (not cold water) and soap, it removes oils from the hands that may harbor micro-organisms.
3. Your hands should first be wet with water, then lather your hands with soap.
4. Your hands should be rubbed together with the soap for about 20 seconds or more, scrubbing the back of your hands, under your nails and between your fingers.
5. Rinse your hands with water and use air or a clean towel to dry.

Using Hand Sanitizers Effectively

There are two things to note when using hand sanitizer. First, it needs to be rubbed into your skin until your hands become dry. Secondly, if your hands are greasy or dirty, it needs to be washed with soap and water before applying hand sanitizer.

With that in mind, the below tips are how to use hand sanitizers effectively.

1. Apply enough sanitizer to the palm of one hand.
2. Rub your hands together thoroughly, making sure that the entire surface of your hands, the back of your hands, under your nails and between your fingers are well covered.
3. Keep rubbing for about 30 to 60 seconds or until your hands become dry. Most times, it takes about 60 seconds and, in other cases, a little longer for the hand sanitizer to kill most germs.

Conclusion

Congratulations on having to transit the lines of this book from start to finish.

In this book, I have provided you with the most valid information that you need to safely make your own hand sanitizer in 5 minutes amidst the scarcity and overpriced hand sanitizers out there in several online stores, supermarkets, and pharmacies. Not only that, but I have also ensured the recipes shared are compliant with the recommended alcohol concentration that is very effective in destroying most bacteria and viruses, including the COVID-19 virus. The preparation process has also been simplified to make it easy for you to understand and follow through with. Lastly, I have shared important tips you need in practicing hand hygiene, which is all but essential toward combating bacteria and viruses. Therefore, it is my sincere desire that you found great value from the invaluable and simplified insights shared in this book, which I hope you put into action right away.

Given the current global pandemic, I urge you to take full responsibility for your overall health and wellbeing.

I wish you the very best on your journey toward a hygienic lifestyle.

References

Lindberg, S. (2020, March 23). How to Make Your Own Hand Sanitizer. Retrieved from https://www.healthline.com/health/how-to-make-hand-sanitizer#effectiveness

Rogers, K. (2019, August 22). Hand sanitizer. Retrieved from https://www.britannica.com/topic/hand-sanitizer

Post, T. J. (2020, March 15). COVID-19: Not all hand sanitizers work against it – here's what you should use. Retrieved from https://www.thejakartapost.com/life/2020/03/15/covid-19-not-all-hand-sanitizers-work-against-it-heres-what-you-should-use.html

Jacobs, K. L. (2020, March 31). Hand Sanitizer (WHO Formula) –. Retrieved from https://www.agardenforthehouse.com/2020/03/hand-sanitizer-who-formula/

Hein, A. (2020, March 17). Coronavirus panic buying prompts DIY hand sanitizer: Avoid mixing these ingredients. Retrieved from https://www.foxnews.com/health/coronavirus-panic-buying-diy-hand-sanitizer-avoid-mixing-ingredients

Marr, K. (2020, March 19). Homemade Hand Sanitizer Spray (Kid-Friendly). Retrieved from https://livesimply.me/homemade-hand-sanitizer-spray-kid-friendly/

A. (2020, April 6). Homemade Hand Sanitizer for Travel. Retrieved from https://52perfectdays.com/articles/homemade-hand-sanitizer-for-travel/

Meagan Visser. (2020, March 14). Homemade Essential Oil Hand Sanitizer Recipes For Adults & Children. Retrieved from https://www.growingupherbal.com/homemade-essential-oil-hand-sanitizer/

Miller, K. (2020, March 14). Does Witch Hazel Kill Germs? Here's Why It's Not Reliable, According to Doctors. Retrieved from https://www.prevention.com/health/a31344840/does-witch-hazel-kill-germs/

Show Me the Science – When & How to Use Hand Sanitizer in Community Settings. (2020, March 3). Retrieved from https://www.cdc.gov/handwashing/show-me-the-science-hand-sanitizer.html